Flávia Rosa Agapito
Ma. Filomena N. Spinelli

Physiotherapy in the Universe of Older People with Intellectual Disabilities

Flávia Rosa Agapito
Ma. Filomena N. Spinelli

Physiotherapy in the Universe of Older People with Intellectual Disabilities

A Systematic Literature Review

ScienciaScripts

Imprint
Any brand names and product names mentioned in this book are subject to trademark, brand or patent protection and are trademarks or registered trademarks of their respective holders. The use of brand names, product names, common names, trade names, product descriptions etc. even without a particular marking in this work is in no way to be construed to mean that such names may be regarded as unrestricted in respect of trademark and brand protection legislation and could thus be used by anyone.

Cover image: www.ingimage.com

This book is a translation from the original published under ISBN 978-3-330-19899-9.

Publisher:
Sciencia Scripts
is a trademark of
Dodo Books Indian Ocean Ltd. and OmniScriptum S.R.L publishing group

120 High Road, East Finchley, London, N2 9ED, United Kingdom
Str. Armeneasca 28/1, office 1, Chisinau MD-2012, Republic of Moldova, Europe
Printed at: see last page
ISBN: 978-620-8-25651-7

Presentation

Writing about ageing is actually looking at a topic that is current and relevant, but which needs extra attention, especially in countries like Brazil that seek to integrate the elderly into the society in which they live, without worrying too much about proposals that would truly make this inclusion possible.

A long time ago there was no possibility of extending the discussion of senescence to those who were always left on the sidelines or labeled and specified as sick - people with intellectual disabilities. As the years go by and scientific advances are made, it can be seen that this population is also increasing its life expectancy, thus fostering the need for scientific studies that shed light on the best way for these individuals to experience this later stage of life.

In this sense, it is essential to understand physiotherapy and its scope in terms of the intersection between these two areas - the health of the elderly and the health of people with disabilities. In this way, the aim is not to present the reader with a ready-made formula of activities to be applied, as this would be disrespectful of people's individuality, but with strategies and paths that can make them realize the importance of working on movement and its various nuances at all stages of life.

What can often seem like an immeasurable challenge becomes motivating and stimulating, to awaken in these people with intellectual limitations and their families the concept of active and participatory ageing, capable of enabling real inclusion.

Maria Filomena Nobrega Spinelli

INDICE

Chapter 1

The most modern thing there is in life is getting old.

(Arnaldo Antunes)

In this chapter, we have tried to characterize, in general and specific terms, the changes resulting from the ageing process, according to the main scholars in the field. What guided and underpinned the research was the real need to know a little more about a phenomenon that in recent decades has attracted the attention of researchers around the world - the demographic explosion of the elderly population.

General Characteristics of the Human Ageing Process

Aging is a biological process, inherent to the human being, which gradually takes place with a decrease in physical strength and vigor due to physiological transformations. The anatomical and functional changes brought about by ageing are not caused by disease and come in different forms, as individual manifestations. However, ageing should not only be understood as an intrinsic process, but also as a biopsychosocial phenomenon, which not only alters the human situation, but also their relationship with the world and their history, bringing psychological consequences, as well as transforming their social and cultural context. Therefore, old age must be fully understood (ABREU, BRUNELLI E TRINDADE, 2005; FREITAS *et al.,* 2010).

Human aging occurs indiscriminately in all human beings, regardless of race, religion, customs or gender, gradually and irreversibly. The aging process involves molecular disorders that affect the cells of vital organs at an undefined point in adult life, in a different dynamic for each person, influenced by the environment, lifestyle, economic and socio-cultural factors. This phenomenon happens to everyone and there is no way of preventing it (PEREIRA, 2011; FECHINE E TROMPIERI, 2012).

Curiati, Kasai and Nobrega (2011) state that there are differences in aging and that the natural aging process is called senescence, composed of a sequence of morphological and functional changes that occur over the years, and is not considered a disease. Senility is considered the opposite, and is seen as the result of damage to the body's health as it ages, caused by bad lifestyle habits and illnesses, and is therefore classified as pathological ageing.

The physical, cognitive and behavioral deficits seen in physiological aging are the result of biological disturbances that cause a series of molecular and cellular events producing apoptosis, protein alterations, the release of free radicals and various other secondary damages. This damage alters the body's systems, occurring at cardiovascular, respiratory, central nervous, peripheral and musculoskeletal levels (SANTOS, ANDRADE AND BUENO, 2009).

Table 1, highlighted below, shows the main systems affected by physiological ageing. The repercussions of each condition and the intensity with which it occurs depend on individual issues, such as the existence of comorbidities, which differs from the natural organic process of a slow and gradual decrease in organ function, which, as previously mentioned by Curiati, Kasai and Nobrega (2011), is usually referred to as pathological ageing or senility.

As these systems are interconnected, the initial involvement of just one of them, if not treated properly, can lead to secondary problems or even worsen initially mild conditions, contributing to further generalized organ decline.

Table 1. Main systems affected by physiological ageing

Cardiovascular	Respiratory	Nervous System Central and Peripheral	Musculoskeletal
- Reduced cardiac mechanics. - Hypertrophy and dilatation of the left ventricle - Stiffness of the arterial walls	- Lung volumes and capacities decrease. - Rigidity of the thorax - Distension of the lungs.	- Decrease in the production of essential proteins - Decreased transmission of nerve impulses	- Loss of mass muscle. - Decreased bone resorption. - Overall loss of muscle strength.

Source: Prepared by the author

Dias *et al* (2012) explain that the ageing process brings with it a higher incidence of cardiovascular disease, associated with a sedentary lifestyle and poor eating habits, which cause various alterations such as a reduction in cardiac mechanics, hypertrophy and dilation of the left ventricle and an increase in the stiffness of the artery walls. Together, these factors are related to the onset of hypertension, heart failure and coronary artery disease. Mello, Fontana and Torrejais (2008) also point out that menopausal women who don't take hormone replacement are more prone to hypertension and, consequently, cardiovascular disease, for reasons such as diabetes, smoking, a sedentary lifestyle and, above all, a lack of oestrogen.

The changes that occur in the respiratory system happen slowly but continuously from the age of 25. Lung volume and ventilation capacity decrease due to the stiffness of the thorax and distension of the lungs, reducing the efficiency of the elastic fibers to return to their original size after inhalation. Early fatigue is observed in the elderly, due to less productive activity, leading to a greater accumulation of blood lactate. This acidosis is consequently compensated for by an increase in ventilatory work in order to expel more carbon dioxide (BRUNELLI, TRINDADE E ABREU, 2005; PEREIRA, 2011).

Brito *et al* (2005) point out that, as age progresses, there is a significant change in respiratory drive, with a considerable decrease in central nervous activity and neuronal impulses to the respiratory muscles, which leads to a minimal response to hypoxia and hypercapnia, explaining that all these changes are present from the age of 50, but are better seen in healthy elderly people from the age of 80.

According to Ricardo, Alves and Meira (2009), during the ageing process there are also changes in the sensory organs or sense organs, which enable us to interact with the environment. In relation to vision, on average, from the age of 60 there is a reduction in the pupil, leading to a reduction in peripheral and night vision and an increase in sensitivity to bright light. Hearing loss in the elderly is not always caused by advancing age, but also by exposure to loud noises and adverse drug reactions. These losses can be conductive, where a series of deformations lead to calcification and increased rigidity of the tympano-ossicular chain; sensorineural, where there is loss of the hair cells of the organ of Corti, neurons, as well as atrophy of the stria vascularis and mechanical transformations in the basilar membrane.

The same authors also report that hearing loss is considered to be the most incapacitating of the sensory organs, since it jointly causes alterations in speech perception, leading the elderly to social isolation.

According to Lima (2007), smell and taste are associated senses and the loss of these senses causes a series of problems for the elderly, such as the consumption of inappropriate and harmful foods with excessive salt and sugar.

Similarly, tactile senses diminish over the years, reducing the ability to recognize the shape and size of objects, as well as the temperature in contact with the body. It should also be noted that touch is very important for locating and positioning the body, physical protection, affection and sex.

With regard to the cognitive abilities of the elderly, Bezerra *et al* (2016) explain that the changes generated by the nervous system due to aging can be neuroanatomical, where there is a loss of brain volume, neurophysiological, when it happens due to a drop in the number of neurons, in addition to a reduction in the competence of synaptic connections and neurochemical with a decrease in the concentration of neurotransmitters, such as dopamine. These deficits lead to a series of problems such as memory loss, plus the effort to control and deal with visual and spatial messages, perform several tasks simultaneously and find the right word to make a subject coherent.

Amnestic Mild Cognitive Impairment (amnestic MCI) is frequently observed in the elderly, as stated by Zanini (2010), as well as early stages of dementia and depression, which need to be seriously assessed so that they are not confused. Dementia is a syndrome in which there is a decline in memory associated with a deficiency in another cognitive area such as executive functions and language that impairs the quality of life of the elderly. There are several types of dementia that affect the elderly, however, Alzheimer's disease is the most prevalent.

With advancing age, there are changes in the quantity and quality of sleep, as reported by Fernandes, Magalhaes and Antao (2012). In general, the elderly sleep less, 6 hours on average, with a longer latency period and a shortage of deep sleep, resulting in non-restorative sleep and an increase in daytime naps, which has repercussions for their quality of life.

1.1 Changes in Functional Capacity

Meireles *et al* (2010) recognize that one of the most significant milestones in the aging process is the functional capacity of the individual, where strength, balance, motor coordination and flexibility are variables that are linked by neurological and muscular alterations. The Central Nervous System (CNS) and the Peripheral Nervous System (PNS) differ in their anatomy, but share a common factor, neuronal aging, where the lack of production of structural proteins, enzymes and neurotrophic factors has a negative impact, making neurogenesis, plasticity, conduction and transmission of nerve impulses more laborious, thus resulting in deficits in static and dynamic balance.

Functional alterations also occur due to deficiencies in the muscular, osseous and articular systems, with a decrease in the volume of white fibers and red fibers. There is a reduction in the number of fibers, leading to a loss of muscle mass, which is replaced by fat, known as sarcopenia. In the bones of the elderly, changes occur in both the cancellous bone and the compact bone. The cancellous bone loses bone laminae, while the compact bone reduces its thickness, reducing bone resorption. As the joint system ages, fibrous tissue is replaced by bone, reducing its resistance to fractures, as happens with the bones of the skull. The decrease in the number and activity of osteocytes leads to a shortage of calcium metabolism, resulting in a significant loss of matrix. This loss is usually more intense in women during the menopause (BRUNELI, TRINDADE E ABREU, 2005).

These musculoskeletal alterations will have an important impact on the posture of the elderly, according to Ferreira and Marquez (2013), who argue that mechanical stress has a negative effect on connective tissue, muscles and joints, causing poor body alignment, failure to distribute loads and pressures on the joints, resulting in inappropriate postures typical of the elderly, such as an anteriorized head, increased thoracic kyphosis and decreased lumbar lordosis, pelvic retroversion and exacerbation of knee angulation and positioning. These are compensatory positions typical of ageing, which in women can intensify in the post-menopausal period.

Alouche and Silva (2013) confirm that the overall loss of muscle strength, the decline of motor neurons and aerobic fitness disrupt the efficiency of walking in the elderly. When they walk normally, they expend more energy and consume more oxygen than young people over the same distance. This is due to increased neural activity, activation and association of sensory areas such as vision and hearing, and modification of automatic control for an intentional effort, when the elderly need to think, correct and redirect their gait.

And despite all the losses observed during ageing, the elderly need to take an assertive and resilient stance, taking advantage of and recognizing their potential and the experience acquired over the years. In this way, Moraes, Moraes and Lima (2007) state that maturing is not just a question of ageing itself, but also of each individual's ability to seek out and give meaning to their own existence. For Fechine and Trompieri (2007), the losses and gains caused during the ageing process are felt in a particular way by each elderly person, produced by educational and cultural factors, but which generally bring doubts and frustrations about their new role in society, economic losses, low self-esteem and depression.

Aging is not synonymous with getting sick, but it does lead to an increase in health care and the improvement of intergenerational relationships. And in order to achieve the much-desired healthy old age, a new approach is needed, which must take into account all of the person's needs, be they biomedical, social, cultural or familial (LITVOC E BRITO, 2004; FREITAS *et al.*, 2010).

Chapter 2

> *Everyone is a genius. But if you judge a fish by its ability to climb trees, it will spend its whole life feeling stupid.*
>
> (Albert Einstein)

The aim of this chapter was initially to clarify the peculiarities of intellectual disability within the context of disabilities in general, and then to explain the aging process of these people, differentiating it in relation to people who do not have intellectual limitations.

ELDERLY PEOPLE WITH INTELLECTUAL DISABILITIES

2.1A QUESTION OF DISABILITY

According to the United Nations (UN) Convention and the criteria of the International Classification of Functioning (ICF), the definition of disability is any impairment or imbalance of an anatomical, physiological or psychological conformation or function that causes incapacity for the proper functioning of a practice that is considered normal for the human being. People with disabilities are those who have long-term physical, mental, intellectual or sensory impairments and various obstacles can prevent them from participating fully in society if they are not given the same opportunities as other people (BATISTELLA, SD).

Bernardes *et al* (2009) and Pfahl (2014) also explain that people with disabilities make up a large contingent of the world's population. It is estimated that there are currently more than 600 million people with some kind of disability in the world, 80% of whom live in developing countries, in situations of poverty.

Oliveira (2012) reports that data from the last census carried out by the Brazilian Institute of Geography and Statistics (IBGE) in 2010 shows that 23% of the Brazilian population has some kind of disability, whether hearing, visual, motor, mental or intellectual, of which 26.5% are women and 21.2% are men. The author also mentions that various types of disability change in relation to people's age and that in the entire sample of disabilities, the highest incidence is in the population over 65. He also points out that, especially when it comes to mental or intellectual disability, this was found in 1.40% of the elderly population.

The life expectancy of people with disabilities at the beginning of the 20th century was around 20/30 years, but recent studies show that this age is currently between 70/80 for the general population (CARRASCO, 2013).

In addition, the same author points out that the term disability requires a biopsychosocial questioning, where variables such as organic, social and psychological conditions have repercussions for the person, their family and society in general. In this way, people with disabilities need to be treated in a preventive and rehabilitative way, but also by investing in their social participation in order to better accept their condition and always promote inclusion.

2.2INTELLECTUAL DISABILITY

With regard to intellectual disability, the American Association on Intellectual Developmental Disabilities (AAIDD) defines it as corresponding to below average intellectual performance, together with adaptive restrictions in two or more areas of competence, such as communication, leisure, work, academic activities, which appear before the age of 18. However, analyzing intellectual disability is not just a matter of scoring below the average (100) on intelligence quotient (IQ) tests, but rather the individual's ability to perform tasks independently despite general incompetence, excluding sensorimotor, visual, auditory and language disorders, as well as other cognitive disabilities. In the hypothesis that an IQ below 70 and good social adaptation, with school and professional aptitude, are proven, it can be confirmed that the low IQ was a false positive result (DALGALARRONDO, 2008; ROWLAND and PEDLEY, 2011).

Rosa (2015) refers to intellectual disability (ID) as a delay in neuropsychomotor development, which can occur in isolation or associated with malformations, neurological symptoms, behavioral disorders and seizures, **and** is a major and profound social problem in the world. Schuck (2012) emphasizes that 3% of the population is affected by ID, making it the most prevalent neurological condition, second only to cerebral palsy and epilepsy. And even with the significant advances in neurology, many patients remain undiagnosed

Dalgalarrondo (2008) explains that intelligence is difficult to define, but it can be explained as the end result of various intellectual processes, in which the individual is able to recognize and solve new problems, as well as identify a complex situation and adopt measures to change it without harm to themselves and within the socio-cultural pattern in which they are inserted. The mental processes that create and organize these chains of reasoning are not innate, as they change throughout human development. He also points out that the area of the prefrontal cortex, considered the executive center of the brain, is myelinated in the period between the third month of life and the beginning of adulthood, reporting that problems occurring in this period may contribute to mental deficits, since the myelin sheath enables more effective and faster neuronal conduction, intensifying brain functions.

Zuna (2012) points out that, around the 1980s, Howard Gardner established the theory of multiple intelligences, which aimed to undo the theory of a single intelligence and establish how vast and diverse mental capacity is, thus constituting 8 types of intelligences, namely: linguistic intelligence, spatial intelligence, logico-mathematical intelligence, musical intelligence, kinesthetic/corporeal intelligence, interpersonal intelligence, intrapersonal intelligence and naturalistic intelligence, also considering that the success of these intelligences varies from individual to individual, depending on the stimulus received and the environment in which they are inserted.

Environmental factors therefore prove to be an important condition for children's intellectual development, according to Rabelo and Rose (2015). Neurologically, childhood is considered to be a delicate stage for cortical improvement, which will depend on the quantity and quality of stimulation of the nervous system through the child's experiences.

Pfhal (2014) also emphasizes that the brain not only adapts to challenging and stimulating conditions, but that it is also influenced by unpleasant and destructive social environments, reinforcing that education and work are important tools in making individuals more intelligent or less competent.

The etiology of intellectual disability in clinically assessed patients is undetermined in 30 to 40% of cases. The causes of the disability can be primary or psychosocial. Among the most commonly found predisposing factors are heredity, such as inborn errors of metabolism, chromosomal aberrations, such as Down's Syndrome and Fragile X Syndrome, alterations in embryonic development, as well as damage in the prenatal period, alcohol and drug use by the mother, peri-natal problems such as prematurity, infections and trauma. In addition to these, other cognitive alterations such as autism are among the possible causes of intellectual disability. Deprivation of affection and care, lack of social and educational stimulation also corroborate a possible cause (DALGALARRONDO, 2008).

According to Carrasco (2013), the male gender is the most affected by intellectual disability, with 100 women for every 116 men. There is agreement among researchers regarding the male sex, because as Vasconcelos (2004) mentions, the various gene mutations are found on the X chromosome.

According to the same author, Fragile X Syndrome is a highly prevalent hereditary cause of intellectual disability, caused by a mutation in the FMR1 gene located at the Xq27.3 locus. The FMR1 gene encodes the FMRP protein, which binds to mRNA, and its transcription-translation regulating effect is indispensable in the maturation and function of synapses. In the normal population, CGG repeats range from 6 to 54 units, while those with the syndrome show an increase of over 200 units, thus establishing the full mutation. A number of CGG repeats greater than 200 implies hypermethylation of the segment, omitting transcription of the FMR1 gene, so the FMRP protein is absent. Populations with 55 to 200 repeats are classified as carriers of the premutation, which is unstable in nature and usually increases during the first female meiotic division.

On physical examination, children with the syndrome have elongated ears and face, may present macrocephaly, hyperextensive joints, hand tremor, hyperactivity and autistic behavior (VASCONCELOS, 2004).

When it comes to motor behavior, people with intellectual disabilities have a lack of balance and locomotion, often presenting alterations in the spine, flat feet, irregularity in muscle tone, thus delaying their neuropsychomotor development.

The most prevalent condition for intellectual disability is trisomy 21, or Down's Syndrome, which, according to research, currently affects approximately 730 babies born in the United States and one in every 800 in Brazil. It occurs as a result of an extra copy of chromosome 21, causing a noticeable clinical manifestation (phenotype) involving facial and musculoskeletal characteristics, a high risk of some types of pathology, such as congenital heart failure, leukemia in childhood, Alzheimer's disease in old age, as well as intellectual impairment, although there are variations between those affected (SILVERMAN, 2015).

Monteiro and Kock (2014) point out that in the last two decades there have been several advances in neuroscience to understand how the human brain works in cases of autism, schizophrenia and intellectual disability. Amaro (2007) reports on a study carried out with 150 children with IQs below 70, for electroencephalographic and magnetic resonance analysis, where it was revealed that 50% of the children had various lesions observed on magnetic resonance, while the other 50% had preserved brain structures, exposing the complexity of this disability, showing that the causes of ID must be structural or functional in terms of neurons and axons and also recognizing biological or cultural family inheritance.

Throughout history, there have been many ways of looking at people with intellectual disabilities, as Garghetti, Medeiros and Nuernberg (2013) admit, ranging from mysticism to extermination, with these people sometimes seen as gods and sometimes as cursed. There have been many expressions used to describe people with intellectual disabilities, such as idiot, imbecile, oligophrenic, exceptional, retarded and mentally handicapped. These terms were left aside whenever other concepts and currents of researchers emerged who were able to explain and understand them in a different way, reaching the present day where intellectual disability is the most appropriate term defined by the *American Association on Mental Retardation* (2006), now called, according to Pletsch and Damasceno (2011), the International Association for the Scientificof Intellectual Disabilities (IASSID). It should also be noted that intellectual disability is characterized by taking into account at least four aspects: biomedical, behavioural, social and educational.

The authors Dalgalarrondo (2008); Girard, Portella and Colussi (2012) state that intellectual disability should not be confused with mental illness, since deficits in problem-solving and social judgment are due to cognitive disabilities and not to thought disorders, as happens in those with mental disorders. There is no one attribute that defines the personality, behavior and physical characteristics of people with intellectual disabilities. Some are passive and dependent, while others are aggressive due to their lack of communication skills. That's why it's so important to know the clinical and functional peculiarities of intellectual disability, in order to understand the manners and attitudes of these people.

Table 2 below classifies the degrees of intellectual disability, intellectual quotient (IQ), equivalent mental age, percentage of individuals affected by intellectual disability and associated disorders.

Individuals with mild intellectual disabilities account for around 85% of the population with ID. They can be fully independent in terms of self-care, such as eating, bathing, dressing and controlling their sphincters, as well as skilled in domestic practices, but they may have some difficulties with reading, writing and mathematical problems. Emotional disorders such as depression, anxiety and aggression also occur in children when they recognize themselves as different and excluded by their peers.

Table 2. General Aspects of Mental Retardation

Degree of mental retardation (MR)	**Intellectual Quotient (IQ)**	**Mental Age (corresponding to a child of)**	**Best attainable school level**	**% of total individuals with MR**	**Associated Disorders**
Limitrofe (not RM)	70 a 84	-	Difficulties Only Appear in High School	Not considered RM	Difficulties with school behavior

Mild MRI	50 a 69	9 to 12 years	6th and 7th grade Elementary school	85%	Conduct disorder, Autism
RM Moderate	35 a 49	6 to 9 years	2nd grade	10%	Conduct Disorder, Autism
Severe MRI	20 a 34	3 to 6 years	Can't Attend School	3 a 4 %	Motor and Sensory Deficits
Deep MRI	Below 20	Less than 3 years	Can't Attend School	1 a 2 %	Sensory motor deficits and eplepsy

Source: Dalgalarrondo (2008)

The moderately intellectually disabled make up 10% of the ID population and have impaired school learning, limited to the second year of school, are able to perform simple everyday tasks under supervision, but are unlikely to achieve independence in adulthood. The so-called severely intellectually disabled often do not speak, as their communication skills are extremely impaired, but they can learn a few words, will need constant support and supervision, do not attend school and have various associated neurological and physical problems, representing 3 to 4% of the ID population (DALGALARRONDO, 2008).

According to the same author, intellectual disability in adults is characterized by the inability to carry out simple everyday tasks such as hygiene, personal care, safety and also limitations in the areas of school, work and leisure, causing difficulties in keeping up with a socio-cultural group, as well as behaving as if they were younger.

Among the most significant limitations in individuals with mild intellectual disability are difficulties with abstract and metaphorical thinking, which are thoughts strongly involved in creativity and imagination and which favor the increase of dentritus-axis, provoking new synapses, which makes them important for learning, acquiring new knowledge and memory. In addition, they also have difficulties with categorical thinking, which is the ability to distinguish facts from the real world from those from the imaginary world, such as legends, differentiating people's particularities, noticing the coincidence of names, places and circumstances, and they also have difficulties in planning an action, preventing the consequences and learning from mistakes (OLIVEIRA E AMARAL, SD, MAHONEY, ALVARENGA E ALMEIDA, 2004; DALGALARRONDO, 2008).

Vasconcelos (2004) states that the doctor's primary task when suspecting a person with intellectual disabilities is to take a thorough history, which will include a family history of neurological diseases, an accurate gestational history, including labor and birth, the parents' educational level, consanguinity, a physical examination with measurement of the brain perimeter, skin inspection, neurological examination and a detailed search for congenital anomalies. Neuroradiological examinations should always be carried out, especially in the presence of epilepsy, microcephaly, macrocephaly, spasticity and in the event of a reduction in acquired skills.

According to the same author, neuropsychological tests should be carried out with caution, always taking into account the sociocultural context, educational level and motivational background of the patient, as well as considering other associated illnesses.

When it comes to treatment, there is no concept of cure in relation to the intellectually disabled, but rather of educability, as emphasized by Carneiro (2007), where all the interventions were based on learning and the pedagogical component.

According to Oliveira, Valentim and Silva, (2013) pedagogical assessment should always have school inclusion as its end result, including a dynamic and continuous assessment, where all the learning possibilities of students with intellectual disabilities are observed, where the report will only serve as a reference, and the teacher will be able to point out paths without labels.

Mahoney, Alvarenga and Almeida (2004) point out that the fundamental role of learning lies in the apprehension and identification of motor, cognitive and affective acquisitions. They also point out that the individual's most primitive activity is circular reaction, in which, through motor exercises, they try to reconcile their movements with the objects within their reach through repetition, and for this reason they emphasize the importance of games, play, perception of differences and similarities, memory and concentration, in order to enable a greater vision of the world, of themselves and of others.

The fact that intellectual disability cannot be cured does not mean that treatment should be avoided. On the contrary, people with ID need early intervention, therapy for associated illnesses, and the family will need support and clarification so that they can defend and help the patient (VASCONCELOS, 2004).

Leitao, Lombo and Ferreira (2008) found that physical rehabilitation is of the utmost importance in this population and must be started as early as possible, as children have impediments in reproducing motor patterns, thus interfering negatively with neuroplasticity.

2.3 AGING OF PEOPLE WITH INTELLECTUAL DISABILITIES

Disability and aging is undoubtedly a contemporary issue that deserves pertinent consideration, but Medeiros and Diniz (2004) report that the issue of disability, despite its wide scope, is little discussed in Brazil and that with the aging of the population it is even more present and will deserve the attention not only of welfare organizations, but of all the movements that are fighting for equality so that meaningful public policies can be introduced.

Society, by infantilizing and detailing people with intellectual disabilities, has not shown that they can reach old age, but this reality has changed substantially, as many people with ID already have a life expectancy that exceeds 60 years of age. It is estimated that in the next 10 years this age will be around 72.7 years (PORTELA, COLUSSI AND GIRADI, 2015).

The aging of the intellectually disabled population is a reality and brings with it a series of physical and psychological changes that are evident and accelerated, since these people have a pre-existing biological weakness (CARRASCO, 2013).

Leitao, Lombo and Ferreira (2008) argue that people who age senescently experience mobility alterations in a phlegmatic way throughout old age, but people with ID experience these problems throughout their lives, even more aggravated by premature aging, which is why all their education and rehabilitation must be started as early as possible, as children, because they have impediments in the reproduction of motor patterns, thus interfering negatively in neuroplasticity.

Functional losses and high rates of dementia lead to worsening mobility in elderly people with intellectual disabilities, as confirmed by Guilhoto *et al.* (2014), who also argue that these losses occur around the age of 30 or 40, which is known as early senility. The parameters of cognitive alterations are equivalent to those found in the course of Alzheimer's dementia in the general population. However, research has shown that individuals with intellectual disabilities exhibit worse health conditions than typical individuals of the same age, with early menopause, hearing and visual disorders, diabetes, obesity, decreased walking and swallowing performance, fatigue, musculoskeletal deficiencies, mental and neurological illnesses, anxiety, aggressiveness and apathy.

The same author mentions a longitudinal study carried out in Spain between

2003 and 2008 which showed that people with intellectual disabilities age prematurely due to a lack of stimulation, health promotion programs and poor access to health services.

Souza and France (2012) reveal studies in which people with Down's Syndrome have a lower life expectancy than individuals with non-specific intellectual disabilities, thus concluding that etiology has a major influence on the aging process of people with intellectual disabilities. They also show that individuals with non-specific intellectual disabilities have greater functionality in relation to activities of daily living (ADL) than individuals with cerebral palsy and Down's Syndrome. According to research, gender has an impact on the ageing process. Just as in the general population the female sex has a longer life expectancy, it is no different for people with intellectual disabilities.

A worrying fact, according to the same author, is that despite many health problems, elderly people with intellectual disabilities only seek medical assistance when their illness is at an advanced stage, due to the lack of verbalization and correct understanding of their problem by family members and carers, as well as less access to health services, which are generally of poor quality.

As previously mentioned, Down's Syndrome (DS) is the biggest cause of intellectual disability, and the life expectancy of these people has increased significantly due to family efforts, early stimulation, physical and cognitive rehabilitation throughout their lives. However, aging occurs prematurely, leading to functional and cognitive deficits. High rates of Alzheimer's disease (AD) are seen in people with DS, as it is already known that trisomy 21 is linked to early and intense deposition of the AD precursor protein, beta-amyloid. However, it is a complicated diagnosis, since people with intellectual disabilities have previous cognitive deficits, and dementia is the main problem faced by people with DS as they get older (FONSECA, *ET AL,* 2015).

According to these authors, it is possible to reverse this situation with stimulation and specific care, seeking a higher level of physical and cognitive skills throughout life, as well as social, work, school and leisure integration.

If on the one hand these individuals have a very low cultural, social and intellectual age, on the other hand their ageing process is accelerating, also as a result of the continued use of medication such as neuroleptics and anticonvulsants, which cause secondary health problems such as osteoporosis and alterations in movement, thus contributing to a loss of mobility and muscle strength (PIMENTA 2011; ALVES, 2012).

Pimenta (2011) observes in his studies that conduct disorders are not very common in this population, but psychiatric problems are already evident in 10% of people with intellectual disabilities, caused by biopsychosocial factors, thus leading to behavioral disorders in these elderly people.

These psychiatric problems may be linked to the fact that people with ID who get older have fewer social contacts and a reduced chance of making friends and, above all, engaging in community activities, thus causing social exclusion (SOUZA & FRANCE, 2012).

Unfortunately, elderly people with intellectual disabilities are discriminated against twice, because they are elderly and disabled. In this context, the biggest challenge for health professionals, family members and carers will be to ensure that these individuals are able to live functionally and meaningfully, without assistance and infantilization, despite their restrictions (ALVES, 2012; GIRARDI, PORTELA E COLUSSI, 2012; OLIVEIRA, 2013).

In view of this, it is essential that the elderly person with ID is cared for in an interdisciplinary and global way, that they are assisted in all fields that involve aging, biological, cognitive, functional, emotional, social and cultural, with the main objective of the health team being the prevention and reduction of functional and cognitive problems, with the improvement of the capacities achieved and a better quality of life (APAE-SP).

There are currently no exclusive public policies for people with intellectual disabilities, however these are mentioned in Law n. 13.146 of July 6, 2015, which establishes the Brazilian Law for the Inclusion of People with Disabilities (Statute of People with Disabilities) in article 2, which considers people with disabilities to be those who have physical, mental, intellectual or sensory difficulties, concomitant with other impediments, and who do not participate fully and actively in society on equal terms with other people. This statute guarantees the right to equality and non-discrimination, priority service in public and private organizations, habilitation and rehabilitation, the right to health, education, housing, accessibility, culture, sport, leisure, information and communication (PLANALTO, 2015).

Ordinance no. 199 of January 30, 2014 of the Ministry of Health in the Actions of the National Policy of Comprehensive Care for People with Rare Diseases in its article 12 on the Organization of Care for people with rare diseases includes the intellectually disabled, establishing that they will have care at all levels of health care. However, the reality in Brazil is that philanthropic and non-governmental organizations such as APAE (Association of Parents and Friends of the Exceptional) and the Pestalozzi Association provide clinical care and social support for these disabled people and their families. The APAEAN movement is the largest in Brazil, with more than 2,000 units serving 250,000 people. The care is multi-professional, serving patients of all ages, accompanying them into old age (AMARO, 2007; TOMAZ *et al.* 2014).

CHAPTER 3

You see: the most important thing The beautiful thing about the world is this: people are not always the same, they are not finished yet - but they are always changing. They tune in or out of tune, that's the truth. That's what life has taught me. That's what makes me so happy.

(Guimaraes Rosa)

This chapter seeks to explain all the resources that physiotherapy has at its disposal to work towards preserving and even increasing the functional capacity of elderly people whose intellectual impairment is configured as a disability. It also highlights the importance of coordinated and targeted movement to maintain brain activity and how to exercise the body and mind of the elderly together.

PHYSIOTHERAPY FOR ELDERLY PEOPLE WITH INTELLECTUAL DISABILITIES

3.1PHYSICAL ACTIVITY

The World Health Organization (WHO) has conceptualized physical activity as any bodily movement produced by the locomotor system that results in energy expenditure, examples of which are sports, day-to-day activities, commuting and locomotion (CHAIM, *et al*, 2010).

The practice of regular physical activity can and should be started at any age, and its benefits are recognized in improving the health of people with chronic illnesses, sedentary and elderly people by promoting weight maintenance or weight loss, limiting the recurrence of illnesses, reducing the risk of cardiovascular disease, increasing motor skills, improving sleep and social interaction, thus restoring self-esteem and avoiding the depression that is so common in the elderly. Physical exercise is crucial for the prevention and rehabilitation of motor deficits related to the ageing process, because depending on the type of exercise, flexibility, balance, motor coordination and autonomy for activities of daily living can be gained (CAROMANO, IDE AND KERBAUY, 2006).

Chaim *et al,* 2010 reveal in their research that the practice of physical activity, through systematized, programmed and repeated physical exercise to gain greater physical capacity among the elderly is associated with a lower incidence of chronic degenerative diseases and deaths, in addition, it results in a significant improvement in their quality of life, also pointing out that the problems conferred by the biological aging process are often linked to disuse, muscle atrophy occurs due to sedentary lifestyle.

According to the same author, the practice of physical activity (PA) represents benefits not only in the physical sphere, but also in the social sphere, since these exercises can be practiced in groups, and in the cognitive sphere, since the exercises stimulate and promote new brain connections, in addition to maintaining the skills already acquired. Baiao (2016) also points out that several studies have shown that moderate to intense physical activity improves memory, balance and leads to a lower incidence of falls, as well as reducing depression and lowering blood pressure, levels of *Low Density Lipoproteins* (LDL) and triglycerides in the blood.

Thus, a good quality of life for elderly people with intellectual disabilities should be encouraged throughout their lives, with healthy lifestyle habits, including regular physical activity, a balanced diet, integrative social, educational and leisure practices.

3.2 ADAPTED PHYSICAL ACTIVITY AND PHYSIOTHERAPY

Adapted physical activity, as Morgado (2015) explains, consists of a wide range of activities, sports and games, always decided by the will, interest, abilities and limitations of these people with the aim of promoting health, reducing injuries, socialization and rehabilitation. Adapted physical activity includes all types of sport for all types of disabled people, whatever their motor limitations and regardless of the purpose of the activity, whether recreational, educational or therapeutic.

According to the same author, the importance of physical activity for the entire human organism is well known and widespread, whether in the physical, mental or social spheres, preventing illnesses or reducing their risk. He also reports that physical activity carried out from a very early age by children and young people with disabilities does not guarantee an adult or elderly person free of illnesses, but it certainly reduces the rate of disorders caused by a sedentary lifestyle, such as obesity, hypertension, diabetes and cardiovascular problems. It also shows that adapted physical activity, in addition to bringing benefits in terms of autonomy, functionality and social inclusion, can turn the disabled person into a competitive athlete, even if this is not the initial goal.

The physical activities applied to elderly people with intellectual disabilities have the same benefits and are the same as those applied to elderly people without disabilities, but take into account their particularities and peculiarities. As described by Campeao (SD), the initial activities should not be too long, nor should their explanations. The actions should be organized in a simple way, so that the person only has one answer, requiring less concentration and time, thus preventing them from becoming frustrated when they fail to perform an action or movement. Still according to the same author, for patients with motor impairment who are unable to perform more intense tasks, other milder but no less significant activities are explored, such as sensory activities, where they can experience and discover their environment through touch, auditory stimuli, music and noise, as well as awakening to new sensations and perceptions such as massage and self-massage.

The practice in this population should be aimed at intensifying and encouraging the practice of physical activities and health education about ageing, as Alfieri and Moraes (2008) point out, so that elderly people with ID can have a better understanding of their bodies and the process they are going through.

According to Arlda (2011), there are aspects that positively inspire elderly people with ID to stay in physical exercise programs, one of which is reward, where prizes, songs and medals make this population stay in the proposed activities longer and more often. In addition, other strategies should be adopted for better adherence to physical activity programs, whether recreational, sporting or therapeutic, including low to moderate intensity physical activities so that there is no discomfort, always starting with a walk for example, the prescription of physical exercise should always take into account the age group, as well as the physical type and cognitive level, and the professional should be prepared to modify the pace and type of physical activity whenever necessary, so as to be able to accommodate all the motor skills of elderly people with ID.

Tribess and Junior (2005) emphasize that the prescription of exercises must take into account the individuality and clinical condition of the patient, whether they are sedentary or active, or have some kind of disability or not.

In view of all the information about the benefits of regular physical exercise, Freitas (2005) highlights the importance it has in promoting the quality of life of people with intellectual disabilities, particularly the elderly with intellectual disabilities, so that the more systematized and enriching activities this population can experience, the greater their motor, psychological and social progress will be.

According to Leitao, Lombo and Ferreira (2016), people with ID experience psychomotor impairments from childhood, which makes it necessary for them to have the opportunity to participate in psychomotricity programs as early as possible, with educational and therapeutic approaches for better rehabilitation and development. Initially, psychomotricity was a prescription of psychiatric medicine, but today it has taken on a multidisciplinary dimension with a preventive, educational, re-educational and psychotherapeutic character.

According to the same authors, the main objective of psychomotor therapy is to improve the individual's relationship with his or her context so that he or she can develop his or her potential through sensorimotor experimentation, with tasks that are playful and organized for everyday reality.

Kinesiotherapy has been the most common physiotherapeutic intervention for maintaining functional capacity and the treatment is carried out in a planned and systematic way through therapeutic exercises such as postural, range of motion (ROM), stretching, aerobic, resistance, balance, breathing and relaxation exercises. The physical impairments most often treated with kinesiotherapy are musculoskeletal, neuromuscular and cardiopulmonary (KISNER AND COLBY, 2005).

According to Vale (2005), stretching and range-of-motion exercises are considered rehabilitative and prophylactic, considerably enhancing the working capacity of muscles, tendons and ligaments, benefiting coordination between them, and this balance is very important for maintaining functional independence in the elderly.

The exercises performed through kinesiotherapy should be adapted to the elderly with intellectual disabilities and their demands, with varied proposals in the form of games and dances, aiming to improve gait, posture, balance and coordination (GARCIA *ETAL*, 2016).

Aquatic physiotherapy aims to achieve the same objectives, since water is a medium that, in addition to having beneficial physiological effects on systems such as the musculoskeletal, cardiovascular and respiratory systems, also enables recreation and socialization. In addition, to the therapeutic benefits provided by water heated to around 36 degrees, such as analgesia and reduced impact on the joints, are the restoration of flexibility, coordination and balance, the improvement of orthostatism and gait, muscle strengthening, sensory, proprioceptive and spatial stimulation, since water is a fickle medium that requires straightening reactions, thus improving patients' posture and agility (BIASOLI, MACHADO,2006; SOARES, SACHELLI, 2008; SILVA, LIMA, 2011).

There are many techniques that can be used in the pool, but when it comes to elderly people with intellectual disabilities, the best method will have to be defined by the physiotherapist, taking into account, in addition to the physical difficulties, an approach that is adapted to the cognitive level of each patient or group. These activities can be carried out individually or collectively, in a playful way, but without losing focus on the main objectives: autonomy, functionality and socialization.

Candeloro and Caromano (2007) also point out that a period of adaptation to the aquatic environment is necessary for the elderly to make the most of the program of motor activities in the water.

It is therefore essential that this period of learning is intensified and developed in a playful and stimulating way for elderly people with intellectual disabilities so that there is adherence, continuity and, above all, motor gains.

Santos (2013) points out that the constancy and improvement of movements is the most important thing for motor progress and that playfulness also generates a series of complex and progressive adjustments in motor activity for the elderly, even those with intellectual disabilities, because the body movements, liveliness and emotions experienced in games directly and indirectly benefit gait, balance and posture, as well as satisfaction with their bodies and attitudes.

An important practice that has become a complement to therapeutic conduct is the use of music, which according to Cerdeira, Varela and Aranha, (2017) favors social interaction and increased self-esteem among the elderly. It is widely used in patients with learning difficulties, motor and mental deficits.

According to Garcia et al, (2006), group exercises are currently a very opportune proposal for adherence to treatment and for strengthening the therapist-patient bond, integrating people with the same needs and facilitating interaction. The same author also points out in his work that diversified group activities with dances, music, body activities and the conquest of new knowledge and potential increases the self-esteem of the elderly in general, reducing or overcoming the much feared and common depression among them, thus emphasizing the importance of forming groups, but designed in a way that is compatible with the particularities of each population.

Fernandes (2005) reinforces that physical activities carried out in a continuous, integrative or rehabilitative way for people with intellectual disabilities bring them greater acceptance of their limitations and improved self-esteem, as they feel able to carry out specific tasks and are close and integrated with other people.

3.3 FUNCTIONAL CAPACITY AND INDEPENDENCE

Pinto and Oliveira (2015) reveal that the numbers are growing in relation to the incapacity and dependence of the elderly due to illnesses associated with sedentary lifestyles, leading them to isolate themselves at home, thus resulting in significant functional losses and generating mental disorders.

An elderly person's functional capacity is measured by their ability to carry out the basic tasks of daily living, BADLs, such as hygiene, eating, getting around and activities that provide independence in the home, instrumental activities of daily living (IADLs) such as taking medication at the right time, making a meal, cleaning the house, managing finances and using means of transport. And this autonomy in carrying out BADLs and IADLs is an indicator of independence, which is a factor that brings self-esteem, happiness and a higher quality of life to these elderly people (PINTO E OLIVEIRA, 2015).

Kato (2013) explains that people with ID have cognitive planning difficulties, which reduces their initiative and interest in new activities, so they tend to sit or lie down more, which leads to less autonomy, functional impairment and depression.

In view of the above, it is essential that people with intellectual disabilities who are getting older are motivated and encouraged not to remain idle and sedentary, but to take an active part in their self-care, home and community activities whenever possible, because according to Breitenbach (SD), inactivity creates a major problem for adults with ID who are getting older: obesity, as well as all its systemic repercussions. Leitao, Lombo and Ferreira (2008) also highlight mobility alterations, such as lack of balance and coordination, as they experience locomotor alterations due to their use of psychopharmaceuticals and because they age prematurely and are at greater risk of developing dementias, such as Alzheimer's disease.

According to Martins *et al* (2007), the elderly person with ID who is able to develop self-care and daily activities independently strengthens their self-esteem, which is closely linked to satisfaction and happiness.

3.4PHYSIOTHERAPY FOR THE ELDERLY WITH DISABILITIES

In view of the above, the demographic change and the new epidemiological picture of Brazilian society, the work of health professionals, specifically physiotherapists, will have to adapt to the new scenario. Junior (2010) points out that physiotherapy's work is based on the curative/rehabilitative model and will have to add new skills to its work, such as health promotion and risk reduction, valuing the social and caring for people in an integral way. In addition, physiotherapists must have the co-participation of other health professionals, doctors, psychologists, nutritionists, speech therapists, social workers, as well as professionals from other fields, such as sociologists, historians, statisticians, engineers and educators.

Incorporated into this context, Abreu, Bruneli and Trindade (2005) state that geriatric physiotherapy previously focused its actions on the patient, but today it works effectively to prevent morbidities that may affect an individual or a population, promoting the physical, psychological and social capacities of the elderly, restoring their functional capacity, autonomy, independence and, above all, improving their quality of life, working preferably in collective activities, respecting the individuality of each individual.

Thus, according to Kato (2013), the main objective of physiotherapy intervention in the ageing process of people with intellectual disabilities is to keep them active so that they can maintain their strength, range of motion (ROM), balance and gait. The physiotherapist needs to work with the motivation of these patients, in group activities, helping social interaction, while taking into account personal interests, with playful activities, with the help of music, dance, colors and balls, with a functional purpose, avoiding infantilization and strengthening patient-therapist trust.

Table 3 below shows the main studies proving the effectiveness of physiotherapy intervention in the elderly

Table 3. Studies showing the benefits of physiotherapy intervention in the elderly.

ARTICLE	AUTHOR(S)	YEAR	CONCLUSION
Music therapy for the elderly in the central sertao of Ceara	Cerdeira, Varela and Aranha	2017	Music and dance improve the functional capacity and quality of life of the elderly.
The influence of physiotherapy with balance exercises on the prevention of falls in the elderly	Gomes, *et al.*	2016	Physiotherapy exercises are important for preventing falls by increasing motor coordination and balance, thus promoting health.
The influence of physiotherapy on the cognition of elderly people with Alzheimer's disease	Medeiros, *et al*	2015	That physiotherapy through physical exercise has great power in preserving < alleviating the effects of the dementia process.

The influence of physical activity in the elderly: A comparative study of the levels of autonomy for the performance of ADLs and IADLs among physically active and sedentary elderly people	Borges and Moreira	2009	That a sedentary lifestyle has a negative effect on functional capacity and that physical activity has a positive impact on improving autonomy in the performance of ADLs and IADLs.

Source: Prepared by the author.

A practical study carried out by Mendes *et al,* (2016) with 10 patients over 60 years of age taking part in a group to improve balance with sensorimotor exercises revealed that physiotherapy exercises are very important for preventing falls in the elderly and that they do improve motor coordination, something that is very impaired in elderly people with ID, and balance, reducing the risk of falls and promoting health.

As previously mentioned, as people with intellectual disabilities get older, especially those with Down's syndrome, they are very prone to developing dementia, especially Alzheimer's disease. In this sense, Medeiros *et al* (2015) report the importance of physiotherapeutic intervention, from the initial symptoms to the most advanced stage of the disease, also emphasizing that not only intellectual activity keeps the brain active and that physical activities are of great importance to preserve and alleviate the effects caused by the dementia process.

The type of program for physical activities with the elderly means little, the most important thing is to keep the elderly active, whether in recreational or therapeutic practices, but when it comes to the elderly with intellectual disabilities, exercise programs need to be more organized and orderly so that they can understand the instructions in order to act and correspond to what is required in the most skillful way possible.

A study carried out by Borges and Moreira (2016) looked at the levels of autonomy for practicing ADLs and IADLs among elderly people who practiced physical activity and sedentary elderly people. 48 people took part, aged between 60 and 88 years old.

13 men and 35 women, found that a sedentary lifestyle has a negative impact on their functional capacity, leading them to a greater degree of dependence in their ADLs and IADLs, and that practicing physical activity for long periods of time improves their autonomy, and even elderly people who start activities at a later age experience the same benefits, concluding that physical exercise improves the quality of life of the elderly.

These findings very much apply to elderly people with ID, since sedentary lifestyles among them are a notorious fact, either due to a lack of opportunity to participate in meaningful and relevant exercise programs geared to their needs, or simply because they don't feel motivated or interested in practicing them.

Cerdeira, Varela and Aranha (2017) carried out a study with 30 elderly people aged between 70 and 79, taking into account the importance of music when practicing physical activities. They found that music is an adjunct to physical exercise and that dancing is the body action most practiced by the elderly. They also point out that dancing brings countless benefits to the body, intensifies memorization and motor coordination and that it can also be performed in groups, which favors socialization.

It is considered by the same authors to be an excellent exercise that, together with music, can minimize anxiety, sadness and make physical activity more pleasurable, thus improving endurance and mood and preventing people from abandoning their activities.

Consequently, the physiotherapist must also dedicate himself to the role of educator, where he stimulates behavioral changes, as well as working with the patient's motivation. In this way, the professional needs to get to know their patient, their pathology, their disabilities, but above all their abilities, their potential, so that they can identify which method and technique will best suit a person with an intellectual disability who is getting older, making this elderly person feel encouraged to learn new skills, so that adherence to treatment is greater and constant, and that they have the initiative to make significant changes pertinent to their health (JUNIOR, 2010).

FINAL CONSIDERATIONS

The subject of ageing has long been discussed and commented on by the scientific community and society in general. However, this does not indicate that the elderly are living and experiencing the benefits of the public policies that have been implemented, or that the increase in life expectancy is due to major improvements in public health. It is understood that there have been advances, but they are unable to meet all demands in an equal and universal way. What can be seen is the presence of long-term care institutions, most of them philanthropic, with or without the support of the Unified Health System (SUS) and families, providing important support for the elderly.

Elderly people with intellectual disabilities suffer from the same difficulties, plus the lack of public policies, stimuli and health promotion actions. They are people who are on the margins of society because they are considered incapable and ineffectual, and they experience all kinds of prejudice. These deprivations further aggravate the situation of disability, adding to the physical, mental and social damage.

The literature has shown that physical exercise for elderly people with ID brings benefits that go beyond strengthening muscles, bones and tendons. It improves body perception, promotes self-care, stimulates self-esteem and, above all, social integration, thus avoiding the apathy and depression that are so common in these elderly people.

Kinesiotherapy and hydrokinesiotherapy stand out as the most efficient and safe physiotherapeutic practices for working with elderly people with ID, since the techniques can be used in different ways, conventional, with music, dangas, in a playful way, individually or in groups, in order to emphasize abilities and aim to acquire new skills.

It was found that people with ID who are getting older need to be motivated and encouraged to learn new activities, practice physical exercise, get to know their bodies and how to take care of them efficiently, without assistance. Families need to be encouraged to acquire new knowledge, just as it is essential that health professionals, who are always tied to the disease process, are able to re-evaluate their therapeutic practice and give new meaning to the practice of care.

Physiotherapy intervention rooted in the practice of cure and rehabilitation neglects essential aspects in the prevention of problems, reduction of risks and promotion of health. Physiotherapists will have to reconstruct their form of intervention with the main objective of developing social and human aspects, working together with other professionals, whether from the health sector or not, because people with intellectual disabilities who are getting older require action and care in the biophysical and social spheres.

However, in the face of many studies, both theoretical and practical, which prove the benefits of physiotherapy intervention with physical activity practices for the elderly, there is a scarcity of studies which establish the exclusive relationship between physiotherapy and intellectual disability. The most significant studies on this relationship are mentioned by the constant work and research carried out by APAE, where professionals carry out relevant activities and studies and accompany these people from childhood to ageing.

However, the study did provide a lot of pertinent and necessary information for understanding intellectual disability and the ageing process of people with it, but above all how they behave, what their needs are and their real potential, so that the best care can be provided.

There is still a need for further research into the issue of physiotherapeutic intervention, with a view above all to preventing and promoting the health of these elderly people.

REFERENCES

ABREU, F. **Anatomical and Physiological Changes in Ageing**. In: BRUNELI,C.B.,

TRINDADE, E.D., ABREU, F.M.C. Fisioterapia Geriatrica. Rio de Janeiro: Shape, 2005. p. 46-51.

Flexibility Exercises for the Elderly. In: VALE, R.G.S. Fisioterapia Geriatrica. Rio de Janeiro: Shape, 2005 p.145.

ALFIERI, F.M.; MORAES, M.C.L. **Ageing and Postural Control**. Revista Saude Coletiva, 2008; v.4, n.19, Ed. Bolina, SP; pag. 30-33. Available at:< https://www.researchgate.net/profile/Fabio_Alfieri/publication/26544800_Env elhecimento_e_o_co ntrole_postural/links/0a85e53440b9410774000000.pdf Accessed on September 25, 2016.

AMARO, K.P. **The Treatment of the Mentally Handicapped in Institutions: A critical analysis from Lacanian psychoanalysis**. Postgraduate Program in Psychology 2007. Pontifical Catholic University of Minas Gerais. Available at:< http://www2.pucminas.br/documentos/dissertacoes_keila_pires_amaro.pdf. Accessed on September 5, 2016.

ALVES, P. J. M. **Estudo de Follow-up do Processo de Envelhecimento em Adultos com Deficiencia Mental**. f.66, 2012. Integrated Master's Degree in Psychology, University of Lisbon, Faculty of Psychology, LISBON, 2012. Available at:<http://repositorio.ul.pt/bitstream/10451/6906/1/ulfpie040142tm.pdf>. Accessed on March 30, 2016.

ARLDA, R.M. **Impacto da Atividade Fisica em Pessoas com Deficiencia Intelectual.** Revista DI, n.1, July/December, 2011. Available at:<http://www.isw.com/zeppelini/does/revista_di Accessed on April 26, 2017.

Association of Parents and Friends of the Exceptional of Sao Paulo (APAE SP). **Support for Ageing.** Available at: <http://www.apae.org.br/OQueFazemos/ParaPessoaComDeficienciaIntelectual /DaVidaAdultaAoEn velhecimento/Paginas/default.aspx>. Accessed on January 20, 2016.

BAIAO, D.A.D. **Functional Physical Fitness and Cognitive Performance in Elderly People with Different Levels of Supervised Physical Activity Practice**. Master's Dissertation in Physical Activity, Castelo Branco

Polytechnic Institute - Higher School of Education, Portugal, November, 2016. Available at:<http://hdl.handle.net/10400.11/5483. Accessed on May 3, 2017.

BATTISTELLA, L. R. **Concept of Disability According to the UN Convention and the Criteria of the**
CIF. Secretary of State for the Rights of Persons with Disabilities. Available at:<http://www.desenvolvimento.sp.gov.br/a2sitebox/arquivos/documentos /274.pdf>.
Accessed on March 28, 2016.

BERNARDES, L.C.G.; MAIOR,I.M.M.L.; SPEZIA,C.H.; ARAUJO,T.C.F. **People with Disabilities and Health Policies in Brazil: Bioethical Reflections**. Revista Ciencia e Saude Coletiva, 2009; 14(1): p.31-38. Available at:<http://www.scielo.br/pdf/csc/v14n1/a08v14n1pdf Accessed on September 15, 2016.

BEZERRA, P.K.; RODRIGUES, K.A.; FELIX,K.D.; SOTERO, R.C.; FERREIRA, A.P. **Cognitive Deficit: Proposal of a Primer for Elderly Care**. Revista Brasileira de Pesquisas em Ciencias da Saude, 2016; 3(1), p. 0-10 Brasilia (DF). Available at:<http://www.icesp.br/revistas-eletronicas/index.php/RBPeCS/article/view/65/67 Accessed on March 15, 2017.

BIASOLI, M.C.; MACHADO, C.M.C. **Hidroterapia: Tecnicas e Aplicabilidades nas fungoes rumatologicas**. 2006. Revista Temas de Reumatologia Clinica. v. 7, n.3, June, 2006. Available at:<http://iasolifisioterapia.com.br/publicacoes/TReuma3-06-Hidroterapia.pdf. Accessed on August 13, 2016

BORGES, M.R.D.; MOREIRA, A.K. **Influências da Pratica de Atividades Fisicas na Terceira Idade: Estudo Comparativo dos níveis de Autonomia para o Desempenho nas AVDs e AIVDs entre Idosos Ativos Fisicamente e Idosos Sedentarios**. Motriz, Rio Claro, v.15 n.3 p.562-573, jul./set. 2009. Available at:<http://cac-php.unioeste.br/extensao/unati/arqs/UNATI_14.pdf Accessed on August 16, 2016

BREITENBACH, N. **Parallels in Ageing.** Ageing Portal. Available at: http://www.portaldoenvelhecimento.org.br/acervo/artieop/Geral/artigo2.htm Accessed on August 29, 2016.

BRITTO,R.R., VIEIRA,D.S.R., RODRIGUES, J.M., PRADO, L.F.; PARREIRA, V.F. **Comparison of Breathing Pattern between Healthy Adults and Elderly.** Revista Brasileira de Fisioterapia, v. 9, n.3 , p. 281-287.

Belo Horizonte (MG), 2005. Available at:<http://www.rbf-bjpt.org.br/files/v9n3/v9n3a05.pdf Accessed on March 15, 2017.

CANDELORO, J.M.; CAROMANO, F.A. **Elaboration, Application and Evaluation of an Aquatic Adaptation Teaching Program for the Elderly.** Revista Acta Fisiatrica, 2007, v.14, n.3, p. 170-175. Available at:<http:// www.revistas.usp.br/actafisiatrica/article/view/102827 Accessed on April 17, 2017. CAMPEAO, M.S. **Sports Activities for People with Intellectual Disabilities**. SD. Available at:< http://atividadeparaeducacaoespecial.com/wp-content/uploads/2014/07/ATIVIDADES-ESPORTIVAS-PARA-DM.pdf Accessed on June 26, 2016.

CARNEIRO, M.S.C. **Mental Deficiency as a Social Production: A Discussion Based on the Life Histories of Adults with Down Syndrome**. Thesis postgraduate program in education. Faculty of Education, Federal University of Rio Grande do Sul. Available at:<http://www.lume.ufrgs.br/handle/10183/10829. Accessed on September 29, 2016.

CAROMANO, F. A.; IDE, M.R.; KERBAY, R.R. **Manutengao na Pratica de Exercicios por Idosos**. 2006. Available at:<//http://WWW.scielo.br/pdf/rdps i/v 18n2a13.pdf Accessed on September 15, 2016.

CARRASCO, L.C.C. Evaluation of **Satisfaction with Life in People with Intellectual Disabilities in the Aging Process**. Master's dissertation, Instituto Superior de Ciencias Sociais e Politicas; Universidade de Lisboa, 2013. Available at:
http://www.repository.utl.pt/bitstream/10400.5Z6583Z1/DISSERTACAO%20 DE%20MESTRADO.pd f Accessed on 21/03/2017.

CERDEIRA, D.Q.; VARELLA, D.S.S. **Music Therapy in the Central Sertao of Ceara.** Revista Fisioterapia Brasil, 2017, v.18, n.1, p. 19-28. Available at:< http://www.portalatlanticaeditora.com.br/index.php/fisioterapiabrasil/article/vi ew/751 Accessed April 29, 2017.

CHAIM, J.; YUASCO, D.R.; FERREIRA, C.A.S.; RAMUNDO, M.E. **Regular Practice of Physical Activity and Sedentary Lifestyle: Influence on the Quality of Life of Elderly Women.** Revista Brasileira de Ciencias do Envelhecimento Humano, 2010; v.7.n.2, p. 198-209. Available at:<http://www.seer.upf.br/index.php/rbceh/article/view/445/pdf Accessed on April 12, 2017. DALGALARRONDO, P. **Psychopathologia e Semiologia dos Transtornos Mentais**. Porto Alegre, Artmed, 2 ed., 2008, p.282-289.

DIAS, D.S.; BERNARDES, N.;BRITO, J.O.; CONTI, F.F.; IRIGOYEN, M.C.; RODRIGUES, B.; DE ANGELIS, K. **Impact of Aging on Metabolic and Cardiovascular Dysfunctions in an Experimental Model of Menopause**. Revista Brasileira de Cardiologia, Sao Paulo, p. 392-399, 2012. Available at:<http://www.rbconline.org.br/artigo/impacto-do-envelhecimento-nas-dysfuncoes-metabolicas-e-cardiovasculares-em-modelo-experimental-de-menopausa-impact-of- aging-on-metabolic-and-cardiovascular-dysfunctions-in-an-experimental-model-of/>. Accessed on March 26, 2016.

FECHINE, B.R.A.; TROMPIERI, N. **The Aging Process: The Main Changes that Happen to the Elderly as the Years Go By**. Interscienceplace Revista CientificaInternacional, Rio de Janeiro, v. 1 n. 7, pag.106-132, 2012. Available at: <htpp://www.intercienceplace.org/isp/index.php/isp/article/download/.../251>. Accessed on January 27, 2016.

FERNANDES, A.; MAGALHAES, C.P.; ANTAO,C. **Sleep and Ageing.** X Jornada de Saude Mental no Idoso: Implicates de Saude Mental no Envelhecimento Ativo. Vila Real- Portugal, 2012. Available at: <http://www.bibliotecadigital.ipb.pt/bitstream/.../sono%20e%20envelhecimento.pdf Accessed on March 16, 2017.

FILHO, W.J.; KIKUCHI, E.L. **Senescence and Senility**. In: CURIATI, J.A.E., KASAI, J.Y.T., NOBREGA, T.C.M. Geriatria e Gerontologia Basicas. Rio de Janeiro: Elsevier, 2011, page 11.

FONSECA, L.M.; NAVATTO, A.C.R. BOTTINO, C.M.C.; MIOTTO, E.C. **Cognitive Rehabilitation of Dementia in Adults with Down Syndrome**. Revista DI, 2015, n.9, p. 17-22 Available: at:<http://upf.br/ser/index.php/rbceh/article/view/2799>. Accessed on April 02, 2017 FREITAS, E.V.; PY, L., CANCADO, F. A. X.; DOLL, J.; GORZONI, M. L. **Physiology of Aging**. In: PEREIRA, S. R. M. Tratado de Geriatria**.** Rio de Janeiro, Guanabara Koogan, 2011 p. 947

FREITAS, M. C.; QUEIROZ, T. A.; SOUZA, J. A. V. **The Meaning of Old Age and the Experience of Growing Old for the Elderly**. Revista Escola Enfermagem USP, Sao Paulo, volume 44 n.02, 2010, p. 407-412. Available at: <https://www.google.com.br/webhp?sourceid=chrome-instant&ion=1&espv=2&ie=UTF-8#q=o%20significado%20de%20envelhecer%20pdf>. Accessed on January 15, 2016.

FREITAS, M.S.S. **Mental Deficiency and Motor Coordination: Comparative Study of Motor Coordination Levels between Individuals with Mild and Moderate Mental Deficiency**. Monograph of the seminar discipline of the re-education and rehabilitation sports option. Porto, December 2005. Available at:<https://repositorio-aberto.up.pt/bitstream/10216/14832/2/6922.pdf. Accessed on October 24, 2016.

GARCIA, M.A.A.; YAGI, G.H.;SOUZA, C.S.;ODONI, A.P.C.;FRIGERIO, R.M.;MERLIN, S.S. **Health Care in Groups from the Perspective of the Elderly.** Revista Latino Am. Enfermagem, 2006, margo/abril; 14(2):175-82. Available at:<http://www.eerp.usp.br/rlae Accessed on August 18, 2016.

GARGHETTI, F.C.;MEDEIROS, J.G.;NUERNBERG, A.H. **Brief History of Intellectual Disability.** Available at:<http://revistareid.net/revista/n10/REIDart6.pdf2013 Accessed on August 24, 2016.

GIRARDI, M.; PORTELLA, M. R.; COLUSSI, E. L., **Aging in the Intellectually Disabled.** Revista Brasileira de Ciencias do Envelhecimento Humano. Passo Fundo, RS, v.9, n.1, p.79-89, 2012. Available at:<http://upf.br/ser/index.php/rbceh/article/view/2799>.Accessed on March 29, 2016. ok

Perceptions of Aging and Old Age among Adults with Intellectual Disabilities. Revista DI, 2015, n. 9, p. 3-10. Available at:<http://upf.br/ser/index.php/rbceh/article/view/2799>. Accessed on April 25, 2017. GUILHOTO, L.M.F.F.; LEONDARIDES, M.R.S.C.; CASTRO, R.L.; SENA, S.; ALVES, A.M.S.; ALMEIDA, C.; KARMELI, D.; MACEDO, E.; TARANDACH, E.R.; RIGHINI, J.B.; PREZIA, M.F.B.; FARIA, V.; CAVALHEIRO, E.A. **O envelhecimento e Deficiencia intelectual na Grande Sao Paulo.** Revista Deficiencia Intelectual, ano 4, n.7,2014, p.5-11.

JUNIOR, J.P.B. **Fisioterapia e Saude Coletiva: Desafios e Novas Responsabilidades Profissionais.** Revista Ciencia Saude Coletiva; v.15, supl.1; Rio de Janeiro; June, 2010. Available at:<http://www.scielo.br/scielo.php?script=sci_arttext&pid=S1413-81232010000700074. Accessed on June 26, 2016.

KISNER,C.;COLBY, L.A.**Therapeutic Exercises Fundamentals and Techniques.** Ed. Manole, 2005, Barueri SP.

LEITAO, A.I.; LOMBO, C.; FERREIRA, C. O **Contributo da**

Psicomotricidade nas Dificuldades Intelectuais e Desenvolvimentais. Revista Diversidades, n. 22, p. 21-24, Oct./Dec., 2008. Available at:< http://www.saberes.com.br/congressoSalto/oficinas/of-3-e-9-/Deficiencia-intelectual-revista%20diversidades_22.pdf#page=21 Accessed October 16, 2016.

LIMA, J.P. **A Influência das Alteracoes Sensoriais na Qualidade de Vida do Idoso**. Revista Cientifica Eletronica de Psicologia, ano 4, n. 8 May 2007; Garga-SP. Available at: <http://www.faef.revista.inf.br/imagens_arquivos/arquivos_dest/sgxfdpcyrrbz4hs_2013-5-10-16- 11-50.pdf Accessed on March 16, 2017.

LITVOK, J.; BRITO, F.C. **Envelhecimento: Prevengao e Promogao de Saude**. Sao Paulo: Atheneu, 2004. p. 226.

MAHONEY, A.; ALVARENGA, A.; RAMALHO, L. **Constituigao da Pessoa na Proposta de Henri Wallon**. Editora Loyola, 2004, Sao Paulo, p. 19-24.

MARTINS, J.J.; BARRA, D.C.C.;SANTOS, M.T.;HINKEL, V.;NASCIMENTO,E.R.P.; ALBUQUERQUE, G.L.; ERDMANN, A.L. **Educação em Saúde como Suporte para a Qualidade de Vida de Grupos da Terceira Idade**. Revista Eletronica de Enfermagem, v. 09, n. 02, p. 443 - 456, 2007. Available at:<http://www.fen.ufg.br/revista/v9/n2/v9n2a12.htm Accessed on July 23, 2016.

MEDEIROS, I.M.P.J.; SECURELLA, F.F.; SANTOS, R.C.C.S.; SILVA, K.M.R. **The Influence of Physiotherapy on the Cognition of Elderly People with Alzheimer's Disease.** Revista Unilus Ensino e Pesquisa, 2015, v.12, n.29, p.15-21. Available at:<http:// revista.unilus.edu.br/index.php/ruep/article/view/686/u2015v12n29e686 Accessed April 21, 2017.

MEDEIROS,M.; DINIZ, D. **Aging and Disability**. Chapter 03; pages 107-120. Available at:<http://www.en.ipea.gov.br/agencia/images/stories/PDFs/livros/Arq_09_Cap_03.pdf. Accessed on October 13, 2016

MEIRELES, A.E.; PEREIRA, L. M. S.; OLIVEIRA, T.G.; CHRISTOFOLETTI, G.; MORAES, M.
R. Q.; SOUZA, D. P. **The Elderly and Disability: An Analysis of the Socio-Affective and Educational Situation of Ageing Students with Intellectual Disability.** Revista Igapo, Amazonas, v.1 p.18-27. Available at: <http://www.ifam.edu.br/cms/images/stories/arquivos/revistaigapo/edicao03/ar

tigo02.pdf>. Accessed on February 24, 2016.

MENDES, M.R.P.; GOMES, A.R.L.; CAMPOS, M.S.; MOUSSA, L. **The Influence of Physiotherapy with Balance Exercises on the Prevention of Falls in the Elderly**. Revista Fisio Senectus, Uno Chapeco 2016, year 4, n. 1, p.4-11. Available at:< https://bell.unochapeco.edu.br/revistas/index.php/fisisenectus/article/view/3299 Accessed April 15, 2017.

MONTEIRO, F.P.;KOK, F. **Exome Sequencing in the Investigation of Intellectual Disability**. Revista Deficiencia Intelectual. Year 4, n.7, July/Dec. 2014. Available at:< http://www.apaesp.org.br/instituto/Documents/Revista%20DI_n7.pdf Accessed August 23, 2016

MORAES, E.N.;MORAES, F.I.;LIMA, S.P.P. **Caracteristicas Biologicas e Psicologicas do Envelhecimento**. Revista Med. 2010, MG; 20(1); pag. 67-73. Available at:<http://www.observatorionacionaldoidoso.fiocruz.br/biblioteca/_artigos/197.pdf Accessed on August 23, 2016

MORGADO, J.M.S. **A Atividade Fisica Adaptada e a Inclusao Escolar dos Alunos com Necessidades Educativas Especiais.** Master's dissertation in Teaching Physical Education in Primary and Secondary Schools. University of Tras Os Montes and Alto Douro, Vila Real, Portugal, Available at:<https://repositorio.utad.pt/bitstream/10348/5909/1/msc_jmsmorgado.pdf Accessed April 01, 2017

OLIVEIRA, A.A.S.; VALENTIM, F.O.D.; SILVA, L.H. Pedagogical Assessment: Focus on Intellectual Disability in an Inclusive Perspective. Oficina Universitaria, Sao Paulo, Cultura Academica, 2013. Available at:<http:// www.marilia.unesp.br/Home/Publicacoes/af-livro_11 oliveira.pdf Accessed on April 18, 2017.

OLIVEIRA, A. F. **Intellectual disability and ageing: A contemporary challenge**. Revista APAE Ciencia, Brashia, v.1 n.1, 2013, p. 33-43. Available at:<http://apaeciencia.org.br/index.php/revista/article/viewFile/4/7>.Accessed on February 25, 2010

OLIVEIRA, J.M.; AMARAL, J.R. **Abstract Thinking**. Available at:<http:// www.cerebromente.org.br/n12/opiniao/pensamento.html Accessed on April 01, 2017.

OLIVEIRA, L.M.B.O. **2010 Census Primer**. People with Disabilities 2012. National Secretariat for the Promotion of the Rights of People with Disabilities. Available at:< http://www.pessoacomdeficiencia.gov.br/app/sites/default/files/publicacoes/cartilha-censo-2010- pessoas-com-deficienciareduzido.pdf Accessed on September 23, 2016 PERRACINI, M. R.; FLO, C. M. **Postura e Envelhecimento**. In: FERREIRA, E. A. G.; MARQUES, A.P. **Funcionalidade e Envelhecimento**, Rio de Janeiro, Guanabara Koogan, 2013, p.154-156.

. FLO, C. M. **Treatment of Dementias in the Elderly.** In: KATO, E.M. **Functionality and Aging**. Rio de Janeiro, Guanabara Koogan, 2013 p. 292-297.

. FLO, C. M. **Gait in the Elderly**. In: ALOUCHE, S.R.; SILVA, L.C.T.O. **Functionality and Aging**. Rio de Janeiro, Guanabara Koogan, 2013, p. 107-114. PFAHL, L. **Inequality, Education and Disability**. Revista Deficiencia Intelectual . Year 4, n.7, July/Dec. 2014. Available at:< http://www.apaesp.org.br/instituto/Documents/Revista%20DI_n7.pdf Accessed on August 23, 2016 PIMENTA, R.L.A. **Necessidades da Pessoa Idosa com Deficiencia Intelectual no Contexto Atual- Reflexoes Sobre a Clinica do Envelhecer: On Needs, Demands, Listening to Desire.** IN: XXIV Congresso Nacional DAS APAES e V Forum Nacional de Autogestao, Autodefesa e Familia, 2011. Electronic Proceedings BELEM, PAG.5-7. Available at:<http://www.itauna.apebrasil.org.br/arquivo.phtml?a=19045>. Accessed on March 30, 2016.

PINTO, F. N. F. R.; OLIVEIRA, D. C. **Functional Capacity and Social Involvement in the Elderly: is there a relationship?** Revista Brasileira de Ciencias do Envelhecimento Humano, Passo Fundo, v.12, n.1. p. 56-68, 2015. Available at:<htpp://www.upf.br/seer/index.php/rbceh/article/viewFile/4687/pdf>. Accessed on June 6, 2016.

PORTELLA,M.R.; COLUSSI, E. L.; GIRARD, M. **Perceptions of Aging and Old Age among Adults with Intellectual Disabilities.** Revista Deficiencia Intelectual, Year 5, number 9, p. 3-10, Available at: <http://www.apesp.or.br/instituto/Documents/DI n.9.pdf>. Accessed on January 20, 2016.

RABELLO, L.Z.;ROSE,J.C. **Is it Possible to Make a Behavioral Analysis of Intelligence?** Brazilian Journal of Behavior Analysis, 2015. University of Sao Carlos SP; v.11, n.1, p. 80-92. Available at:<http://www. periodicos.ufpa.br/index.php/rebac/article/view/2382/3807 Accessed on March 22, 2017

RIBEIRO, L.C.C.; ALVES, P.B.; MEIRA, E.P. **Percepção dos Idosos Sobre as Alterações Fisiológicas do Envelhecimento.** Revista Cienc. Cuid. Saude, v.8, n.2, p. 220-227. Available at: <http://www. periodicos.uem.br/ojs/index.php/CiencCuidSaude/article/view/8202/4929 Accessed on March 25, 2017.

ROSA, M.T.A.S. **Clinical Characterization of Patients with Syndromic Intellectual Disability and Chromosomal and Submicroscopic Alterations Detected by Microarray Chromosomal Analysis**. Dissertation for a master's degree in medical sciences from the University of Brasilia. Available at:< http://repositorio.unb.br/bitstream/10482/18770/3/2015_MariaTeresaAlvesdaSilvaRosa.pdf. Accessed on August 15, 2016.

ROWLAND, L. P.; PEDLEY, T.A., Treatise on Neurology In: **Mental Deficiency.** Rio de Janeiro, Guanabara Koogan, 2011, p. 578.

SANTOS, F. H.; ANDRADE, V. M.; BUENO,O. F. A. **Ageing:** A **Multifactorial Process.** Psicologia em Estudo, Maringa, v.14 n.1 PG.3-10, 2009 Available at: <http://repositorio.unesp.br/bitstream/handle/11449/30216/S1413-73722009000100002.pdf?sequence=1&isAllowed=y> .Accessed on March 28, 2016

SANTOS, S.L. **Effects of a Psychomotricity Program on the Well-being and Gait of the Elderly**. 2013. Master's dissertation Nursing Postgraduate Program, Center for Health Sciences, Federal University of Paraiba. Available at:<http://www.ccs.ufpb.br/ppgeold/dissertacoes2013/sarajlinsdossantos.pdf Accessed on October 25, 2016

SCHUK, P.F. **Erros Inatos do Metabolismo e Deficiencia intelectual**. Revista Deficiencia Intelectual, 2012; n.2; jun/julho, pg. 6-11. Available at:< http://www.apaesp.org.br/instituto/Documents/Revista_DI_n2.pdf Accessed on September 17 2 016.

SILVA, A.S.D.;LIMA, A.P. **The Benefits of Aquatic Rehabilitation for Special Groups.** Available at:<http://www.efdeportes.com/efd160/os-

beneficios-da-reabilitagao-aquatica.htm Accessed on September 28, 2016.
SILVERMAN, W. **Cognitive Characteristics of Down Syndrome**. Revista DI, APAE SP, 2015, n.9, p. 23-29. Available at:<http://www. http://pt.calameo.com/books/001347252a458465518d0 Accessed on 01/05/2017.
SOARES, M.A.; SACHELLI, T. **Efeitos da Cinesioterapia no Equilibrio de Idosos**. Revista Neurociencias, 2008; 16/2: pag. 97-100. Available at:< http://revistaneurociencias.com.br/edicoes/2008/RN%2016%2002/Pages%20from%20neuro_vol_16_ n2-5.pdf Accessed September 26, 2016.
SOUZA, R.D.; FRANCE, V. **Research on the Transition to Adulthood and Aging in the Intellectually Disabled Population.** Revista de psicologia, 2012, n. 1, v. 3, p. 281289. Available at:<http://www. dpc.uevora.pt/.../A%20investigagao%20sobre%20a%20transigao%20para%20a%20v... Accessed on April 26, 2017.
TOMAZ, R.V.V., ROSA, T.L., VAN B. D., MELO, D. G. **Public Health Policies for the Intellectually Disabled in Brazil: An Integrative Review.** Revista Ciencias de Saude Coletiva 21(1): pag. 155-172, 2014. Available at: <http://www.scielosp.org/pdf/csc/v21n1/1413-8123-csc- 21-01-0155.pdf>.Accessed on June 25, 2016 TRIBESS,S.;JUNIOR,J.S.V. **Prescrigao de Exercicios Fisicos para Idosos**. Revista Saude Com, 2005; 1(2);pag 163-172. Available at: <http://www.uesb.br/revista/rsc/v1/v1n2a10.pdf VASCONCELOS, M.M. **Retardo Mental**. Jornal de Pediatria, RJ, v.80, n.2, Suppl. 0, Porto Alegre, April 2004. Available at:<http://www. scielo.br/scielo.php?script=sci_arttext&pid=S0021- 75572004000300010 Accessed on March 29, 2017.
ZANINI,R.S. **Dementia in the Elderly: Neuropsychological Aspects.** Revista Neurociencias 2010; 18(2), p. 220-226. Available at: <http://www.revistaneurociencias.com.br/edicoes/2010/RN1802/262%20revisao.pdf Accessed March 16, 2017.
ZUNA, A.S.C. **Promoting Linguistic Intelligence and Logical-Mathematical Intelligence in Primary School Students.** Master's Degree in Teaching in the Pre-School and Primary School Specialty. Polytechnic Institute of Beja; Portugal 2012. Available at:< http://www.comum.rcaap.pt/bitstream/10400.26/3942/1/Inteligencias%20Multiplas.pdf Accessed on March 15, 2017.

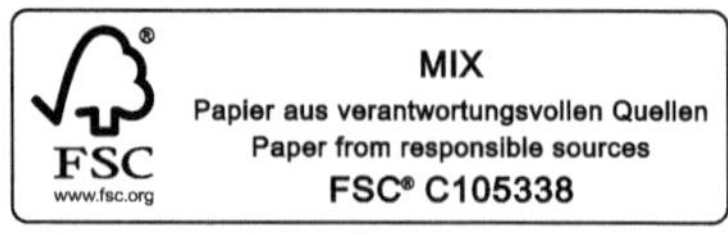

Printed by Books on Demand GmbH, Norderstedt / Germany